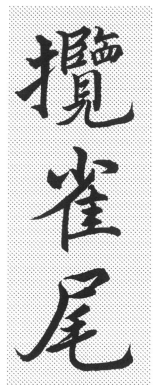

How To

Grasp The Bird's Tail

If You Don't Speak Chinese

BUSINESS, SCIENCE & TECHNOLOGY
QUEENS BOROUGH PUBLIC LIBRARY
89-11 MERRICK BLVD. JAMAICA, NY 11432
(718) 990-0760

Jane Schorre

Calligraphy by Margaret Chang

Arts of China Seminars

Cover: *Mynah Birds, Old Tree and Rock*
Zhuda (c.1626-1705) Qing dynasty
Hanging scroll, ink on satin (204.6 x 54 cm.)
The Nelson-Atkins Museum of Art,
Kansas City, Missouri (Purchase: Nelson Trust)

Text copyright © 1997 by Jane Schorre
Calligraphy copyright © 1997 Margaret Chang

All rights reserved. Address inquiries to:

        Arts of China Seminars
        2314 Driscoll Street
        Houston, Texas 77019

Printed in the United States of America

Publisher's Cataloging-in-Publication
(Provided by Quality Books, Inc.)

Schorre, Jane.
        How to grasp the bird's tail if you don't speak Chinese : a
        light-hearted look at meaning in taiji / by Jane Schorre ; with
        calligraphy by Margaret Chang.   --1st ed.
            p. cm.
        Preassigned LCCN: 97-71308
        ISBN: 0-9657716-0-1

        1. T'ai chi ch'uan--Dictionaries.   I.Title.

GV504.S34 1997   796.8'155'014
                                  QBI97-40637

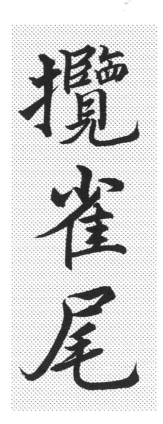

攬雀尾

Contents

Preface

For twenty five years after my introduction to Taiji I worked hard at learning, practicing and teaching it. Only after that was I able to play at Taiji, and only after that was I able to play with the names of the movements as I have in this book. That is the spirit in which it is offered, which is not to say I was not serious in putting it together. For I was serious, in the way that we can be about the games we play.

As we finish up all the loose ends here in order to go to the printer, the 29th anniversary of my first Taiji class approaches. In thinking back over all those years, there are memories of many people whose teachings are reflected in these pages. There are memories of June Yuer and Mary Chow, the teachers who introduced me to Taiji. And there are memories of many years of joyful, playful learning with Chungliang Huang, Jay Goldfarb and The Living Tao. My sincere thanks to them all.

At the same time, the end of almost four years of leisurely play in putting this book together is in sight. Hopefully it will reflect the joy felt in creating it. Many people have been a part of the process, but there are some who merit special thanks. First of all, there is Margaret Chang, whose casual remark sparked this whole endeavor in the first place, and without whose interest it would never have happened. Grateful thanks to Margaret, not only for her beautiful calligraphy, but also for the many hours she spent talking with me about these characters and offering suggestions. And more grateful thanks to her for all the good times we have spent sharing our Taiji experiences. There are Kathryn Davidson and Martin Goldman, who read the manuscript and gave much helpful advice. There are Carrin Dunne and Annette Sanford, my wonderful reader/editors, who helped me get it all together. And there is my husband, Barth, who has given his encouragement and support all along.

"Chinese words are good and bad this way, so many meanings, depending on what you hold in your heart."

Amy Tan
The Hundred Secret Senses

A Beginning

The more I study Taiji, the less I seem to know. Or at least, the more there is to learn. This is really not surprising, considering the many facets of Taiji. It is an exercise for health, a system of self-defense, a method of meditation, an expression of a way of life, a choreography of dance movement, a vehicle for spiritual growth, a path to self-realization, and a celebration of the life force within us – and more. But each of these is only a facet of the whole that is Taiji. In my on-going learning, I find over and over again that each small new discovery tends to open up a whole unexplored territory requiring me to become a beginner again. Along the way I have given up on any dream of ever becoming a master of Taiji, and am hoping instead to someday become a master of beginning. But I find this is what keeps my Taiji forever fresh and absorbing. There is always something new to play with.

An example is the casual observation that finally resulted in this book. It all began one day when my friend, Margaret Chang and I were having lunch together after our Taiji session. She was explaining that, to help her Taiji students get a feel for the movement, she tells them that *An,* usually translated into English as *Push,* is the Chinese verb used for massage, to push into something. And somehow knowing this always changes the quality of their movement, even if only in a very subtle way. This brought up a memory of being told, years ago by a Chinese man, that without understanding Chinese it was impossible to fully understand Taiji because one would never know what the names mean. The man himself is gone from memory, but not his words, in spite of the fact that I dismissed them at the time. I was sure then that any meaning would be in the movement, not in the names. Those were the days when I knew a lot. But I did not know how much our interpretation of meaning in a name can affect the quality of our total Taiji experience. It took the process of this book to begin to learn that.

Margaret's bit of information about *An* set off a small alarm in my head. What else did she know about Taiji that I did not – just because Chinese is her native language? It seemed more than a little unfair she had such an advantage over me. In talking about other names, we realized many of them lose a lot in translation. While often true of any translation, this seems especially true of translation from Chinese, because of its nature, which we will discuss later.

Much in the names of Taiji movements is lost to those of us who, since we do not know Chinese, must rely on the usual English translations. It occured to me that exploring each name for possible meaning might be fun. These names run the gamut from the most poetic to the most prosaic, and from the near sublime to the near ridiculous. Some have to do with profound philosophical subjects, reflecting Daoism and Buddhism. Some suggest ways of deporting oneself, while others suggest only ways of moving. Some are simply the names of everyday objects or are about using objects. Some describe the movements of animals or ways of dealing with animals. Many about kicking or hitting seem to be straightforward descriptions of self-defense movements.

Reactions to the names run as wide a gamut. I am surprised and delighted to find many of them bring to mind stories told in Zuangzi, the Daoist classic second only to Laozi. Some of the Taiji names can evoke a sort of spiritual resonance. Some carry with them a host of associations, while others suggest little more than the obvious, so there seemed to be little to say about them. Some do not seem to make much, if any, sense. Some, in studying them, have changed my feeling about a movement, and therefore changed the way I move.

Eventually, along the way a wonderful game evolved, resulting in this book. It is like a giant puzzle to be taken apart and put back together again, or like a secret code to be broken in order to decipher the message. And imagine my surprise when there actually did seem to be a hidden message in the end!

How To Grasp the Bird's Tail.

In the beginning, Margaret spent many hours with me talking about the Chinese characters and pouring over dictionaries. Then finally the search for meaning led me to my tattered copy of the book by Dr. L. Wieger, S.J., *Chinese Characters, Their origin, etymology, history, classification and signification.* (Dover Publications, 1965). *Chinese Characters* was originally published in French by the Catholic Mission Press in 1915. My Dover edition is a republication of the 1927 edition of the translation by L. Davront, S. J.

Dr. Wieger's book is not as academic and dull as the title sounds. It is scholarly but not stuffy, and occasionally even humorous. Some of the information there is probably outdated now, because of new discoveries and studies in Chinese etymology. But it has been my primary reference because I like it – and because this is only for fun, after all.

The aim here is not to give any definitive meaning of the words or names, but only to explore possible meaning. Letting go of this aim is necessary, because both words and names can be interpreted in many ways and on many levels – at least as many as there are facets to Taiji. Also, the characters used are not always the same. In these cases the differing words are usually pronounced the same, or nearly so, but the written characters have completely different meanings. This suggests that some of the names we use today may not be at all what was originally intended. They may have been passed on orally for many years, with the written word unknown. But this only adds to the enjoyment of the mysterious names and their meaning. Hopefully this enjoyment can be communicated as you follow along with me.

First, to find meaning in a character, we begin by really looking into it to see exactly what is there. Each word is made up of one or more elements, which are something like the building blocks of the language. These are composed of the brushstrokes, which are not at all arbitrary, no matter how they may appear to one who does not know Chinese. Each of these elements indicates a meaning and/or a sound, and can be used alone or in combination to form new words. So, we begin our search for meaning by discovering what elements make up the character.

These elements are always pictorial representations of direct experience. All language may be based on pictures originally, but Chinese has kept them through the millennia. The characters are not words as we know them, but pictures that convey ideas with sounds attached to them. One of the things I enjoy most about Dr. Wieger's book is his clear demonstration of how ancient primitive drawings remain the basis for each character even though it has changed and evolved through time, primarily through changes in writing instruments and styles. This does not mean most Chinese recognize more than a few of the pictures present in the characters, or are often aware of them as they use the words. But the point is the messages are there, and they do affect the use of words and how we respond to them, even if on an unconscious level. This is true of all languages, because the roots of each word are still there. The difference is that in most other languages the immediacy of a visual image is lost in an alphabet system.

Second, after finding the elements that make up the character, we allow our imagination to play with what we discover, with any implication, suggestion, connotation, or symbolization we may find there. Each character is a cluster of associations, of pictorial images of concrete things that resound with metaphoric overtones. The Chinese language is figurative rather than literal and its meanings are implicit rather than explicit. Because of its rich poetic symbolism and its heavy reliance on metaphor to convey meaning, reading Chinese has been called an act of creation.

Our game seems to work best when we keep our minds soft, flexible and flowing – welcoming and enjoying any association that comes along, no matter how fanciful it may seem. After all, this is a game and not a scholarly pursuit. Of course what we find in each character is colored by our own approach to Taiji. My interest in Taiji is not so much in the application as in the spirit of the movements. I do Taiji because I like to, and in doing what I like, I learn a way of being. Each person's individual approach determines the experience of Taiji, as well as the interpretaiion of any meaning discovered in the characters. What I discover here is mine. I invite you to discover your own.

Third, only after exploring the elements of each character and our individual response to them, do we look for dictionary meanings. Please do not focus on them too much. Why? 1.) We have a tendency not even to see the Chinese characters where English is given. 2.) They are themselves translations into English, approaching the meanings in varying degrees. 3.) The very purpose of definitions is to fix or limit. Just look up the word *flower* in any dictionary to see how fixing and limiting definitions can be. 4.) Chinese characters often, perhaps usually, have an inherent ambiguity allowing for multiple interpretations. One meaning doesn't rule out another – even many others. 5.) Hopefully we will be able to see the dictionary meanings as only convenient hooks holding the many associations evoked by the character. 6.) In our exploration, we do not want to come to any conclusions. We want to leave these meanings open-ended, allowing plenty of room both for individual interpretation and for change as we each grow in understanding and experience......For these reasons I was tempted to completely omit the dictionary definitions. But we do need them as sign posts of a sort, after all.

Playing with meaning in the characters and the names, has led me more deeply into my Taiji learning. I feel many new dimensions have been added to my practice of Taiji. I have also developed a profound appreciation for the beauty and poetry of the Chinese language, with its imagery and metaphor creating multiple layers of meaning in each word. And I have enjoyed wandering along the many paths these images have opened up.

If You Don't Speak Chinese

This is a book for meditating – on the characters and their meanings as they relate to the Taiji experience – written for those who know something about Taiji, but little if anything about the Chinese language. Because I know, from experience, how very intimidating these characters can be, this section of the book is offered as a guide to its use.

But first, we have to consider the characters. Most of us in the West have never taken the time to really look at Chinese writing. When confronted with it, we seem to close our vision somehow, not expecting to recognize anything there. This book asks you now to really look at the characters. They are what it is all about. Here, instead of the usual photographs found in Taiji books, of people in various poses, you will find Margaret's calligraphy of the Chinese names. They are there for the enjoyment of their beauty, as well as the exploration of their meanings. At the same time, they can convey a lot about the inner essence of Taiji even though they give no clue to its exterior shape. I hope they will come to life for you.

Like all the arts of China, both Taiji and calligraphy grow out of the ancient, unique Chinese world view of one energy existing in organic yin/yang polarity. The substance of both Taiji and calligraphy is that one energy, chi (or *qi,* in pinyin). In fact, the calligrapher uses a brush as an extension of energy in the same way a Taiji artist uses a weapon: a sword, knife, staff or fan. Both are concerned with the unity, harmony, balance and rhythm of the complementary yin/yang opposites. In calligraphy we see this as brushstrokes held together in a kind of suspended orbit around a center; in Taiji we know it as the whole person moving through space around a center.

The kinship of Taiji and calligraphy is seen in other ways:

1. Calligraphy is, like Taiji, a movement art. What we see as separate brushstrokes in calligraphy are the traces left on paper of one brush stroke moving through space. The brush may circle above the paper for a moment to come back down in another place, but it makes one stroke from beginning to end. In the same way, what we distinguish as separate movements in Taiji are, like a river, one continual flow from beginning to end.

2. Both use fluidity, flexibility and softness to create an expression of strength and power. The soft, flexible brush and fluid ink in calligraphy is a metaphor for the body in Taiji.

3. Like Taiji movement, Chinese characters express the quality of the artist's energy at that moment, flowing from mind through body and revealing the essence of the person. For instance, Margaret's characters are happy, with a deep sense of simplicity, clarity, order and quiet dignity. In the same way, we cannot hide much of ourselves in our Taiji movement.

Chinese characters can be seen as abstract representations of Taiji movement quality. Because of their organic balance, each can be seen as a gesture or a posture of a living thing – a human body or other form of nature. In fact, in them we see the same asymmetrical balance and sense of a brief pause in movement that Taiji photographs have. So I hope you will really look at this Chinese writing and see it for its beauty, its meaning and its relationship with Taiji. To that purpose, the text has been kept to a minimum in order to let the pictures carry the message.

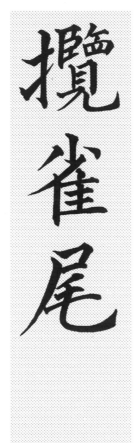

Lan que wei

(lahn chueh way)

Grasp the bird's tail   16

As you turn through the book, you will see on the left hand pages the names of the Taiji movements in calligraphy. Next to these, you will find each name spelled out in pinyin, which is currently the more or less accepted system for alphabetizing the Chinese language. Through the years many different systems have been devised to apply our alphabet to Chinese. But keep in mind these are only keys to the pronunciation of the characters. I use pinyin because it is the system used in China and because it seems to offer better clues to pronunciation (for example Dao instead of Tao).

The fact that I have used pinyin only means you will find familiar names, like Tai Chi, Chuang Tsu, Lao Tsu and I Ching, look like Taiji, Zhuangzi, Laozi and Yijing. This is very confusing if you are not Chinese. Furthermore, unless you have studied pinyin it is as impossible to read as all the other systems created for this purpose. This is very confusing even if you are Chinese.

But please do not give up. Here you have not only the pinyin key to pronunciation, but under that in parentheses, the Jane Schorre key to the pronunciation of the pinyin key to pronunciation! This is given because, even though pinyin is a key to pronunciation, it can't be used as a key until its pronunciation is learned. As I am just trying to learn this myself, I can't make any promises — but if you try reading the words in parentheses while letting the tone of your voice follow the direction of the mark drawn above each syllable, it may even sound a little like Chinese. Good luck!

On the right hand pages you will see:

1. The characters treated separately, with the pinyin for each above it.
2. **In bold type – the dictionary definition.** In regular type – the image meaning. The definition is missing in a few instances where one could not be found. And the image meaning is missing in the few instances where the definition says it all.
3. The component elements of each character. There are usually two primary elements, and occasionally these are broken down further to make it clearer (or more confusing, depending on how you see it). The meaning is usually conveyed very clearly by the concrete images making up these elements. There are times, however, when the dictionary meaning is an abstraction growing out of a concrete image. These dictionary definitions are given in parentheses. Also, in a few instances a primitive character is added for fun and enlightenment.
4. Notes on things that came to mind in playing with the characters. You will find comments about the symbolism, metaphor or allegory I found there, along with some thoughts and feelings about these discoveries. In addition, there are sometimes stories (usually from Zhuangzi) when they seem to be relative somehow.

The original plan was to omit the English translations on these pages, to force you to really look at the Chinese writing. But after several manuscript readers panicked, the translations were added in very small print at the bottom of each page. These are not fixed by any means, for there are often multiple meanings of the words, offering many possible translations. You may come up with some of your own.

This is basically how the game is presented. Have fun!

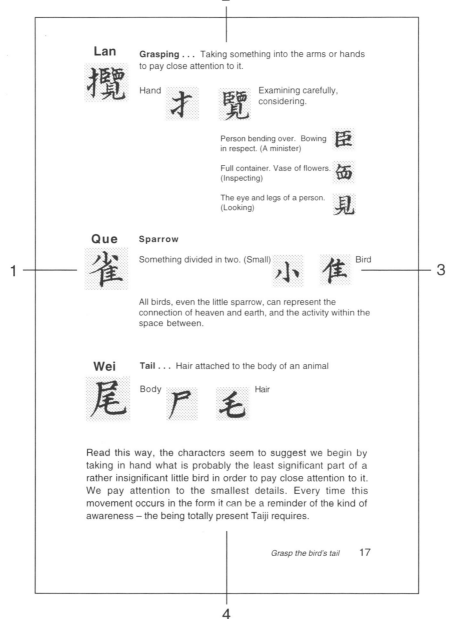

Lan 攬 Grasping . . . Taking something into the arms or hands to pay close attention to it.

Hand 才 覽 Examining carefully, considering.

Person bending over. Bowing in respect. (A minister) 臣

Full container. Vase of flowers. (Inspecting) 缶

The eye and legs of a person. (Looking) 見

Que 雀 Sparrow

Something divided in two. (Small) 小 佳 Bird

All birds, even the little sparrow, can represent the connection of heaven and earth, and the activity within the space between.

Wei 尾 Tail . . . Hair attached to the body of an animal

Body 尸 毛 Hair

Read this way, the characters seem to suggest we begin by taking in hand what is probably the least significant part of a rather insignificant little bird in order to pay close attention to it. We pay attention to the smallest details. Every time this movement occurs in the form it can be a reminder of the kind of awareness – the being totally present Taiji requires.

Grasp the bird's tail 17

11

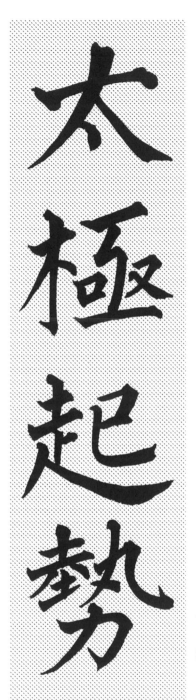

Tai ji qi shi

(tỳ jéé chěe shùh)

Tai

Greatest, highest, most remote. Superlative

Person opening, expanding, growing. (Big, great, old)

Distinguishing mark. Divine spark

Ji

Utmost point. Extreme . . . Polarity. The ultimate union of opposites.

Tree

Heaven and earth connected by the person using mouth and hand. Activity in time and space. (Reaching, coming to. Timely)

Person connecting heaven and earth   Mouth   Hand

Qi

Rising, beginning . . . Self-generated movement.

Person with legs and arms in motion. (Walking, going, traveling)

Self, oneself

Shi

Circumstances. Gesture, aspect . . . Strength required for cultivating the earth.

Sinew, strength   Cultivating the earth. (Skill, ability. Art, craft)

Earth mound   Hand doing something

The characters of *Tai ji qi shi* are loaded with images that can contribute new depth to our experience of Taiji. And, if we enter into them, these simple and concrete images can, through the immediate knowledge of the body, also enhance our experience of the living philosophy at its foundation.

Tai shows a person, already great and still growing, with the gentle warmth of a sacred flame marking the center. Whenever there is a center there is a oneness. As we take our place to prepare for our Taiji practice, we can put ourselves into this image in order to get in touch with our own center and our own unity.

In *Ji* we see first a tree which can represent the world axis. Its roots going down deep in response to earth's gravity provide the tree with stability and nourishment, the gifts of yin/earth. At the same time, its branches are growing toward the light of heaven in such a way that its very form is shaped by that light. This is the gift of yang/heaven. We get a sense of ying/yang polarity which is then augmented by the two horizontal lines in the element to the right of the tree. Between these heaven and earth lines we see the realm of the person, where the eternal balancing of these two primal forces gives rise to our flowing world of space and time. In addition we see a mouth (words, mental abilities) and a hand (deeds, physical abilities) representing spiritual and physical activity in the human realm. In the stillness and silence before we begin to move, we can experience the essence of Taiji in ourselves.

Scholar Reclining and Watching Rising Clouds
Ma Lin (c. 1180 - 1256) Southern Song dyn.
Fan mounted as album leaf, 25.1x25.2 cm.
© The Cleveland Museum of Art, 1996
John L. Severance Fund, 1961.421

In *Qi* we see the person moving, and the self that is the mover. With this image in mind we can be aware of movement arising out of stillness and silence. It just happens. It can come from a source deep within us, so that we move easily, naturally and freely, with a sense of rhythm reflecting the alternating yin/yang current.

And finally, in *Shi* we see a hand working the earth and a muscle tendon. These images can suggest the potter's craft, and there is an analogy there with our Taiji practice. We are the clay as well as the potter. We work the clay to make it flexible and smooth so that it will take the shape we want to give it. We put it on the potter's wheel of Taiji, where mind guides our bodies in realizing the form. It is mind in harmony with body which empowers us to cultivate and create.

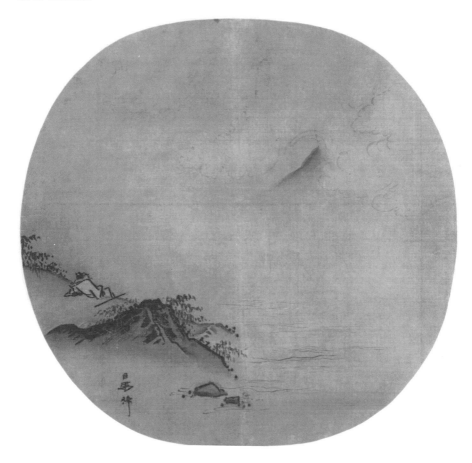

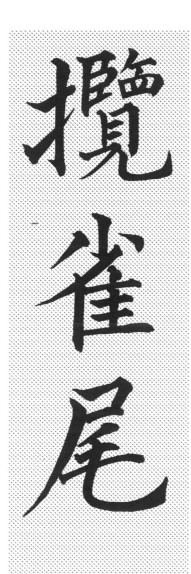

Lan que wei
(lahn chueh way)

Lan

Grasping . . . Taking something into the arms or hands to pay close attention to it.

Hand

 Examining carefully, considering.

Person bending over. Bowing in respect. (A minister)

Full container. Vase of flowers. (Inspecting)

The eye and legs of a person. (Looking)

Que

Sparrow

Something divided in two. (Small)   Bird

All birds, even the little sparrow, can represent the connection of heaven and earth, and the activity within the space between.

Wei

Tail . . . Hair attached to the body of an animal

Body Hair

Read this way, the characters seem to suggest we begin by taking in hand what is probably the least significant part of a rather insignificant little bird in order to pay close attention to it. We pay attention to the smallest details. Every time this movement occurs in the form it can be a reminder of the kind of awareness – the being totally present Taiji requires.

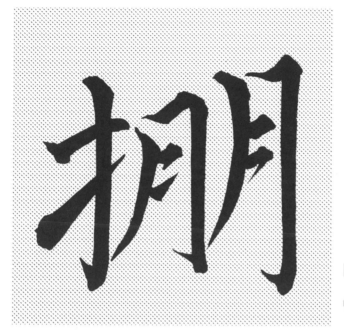

Peng
(púhng)

Peng

Peng is a very obscure word. Even the classical Chinese dictionaries are not clear about its meaning, but suggest it is about expanding and opening up, as well as releasing — about shooting a bow, removing the cover of a container or drawing the cork from a bottle. It also seems to have something to do with the kind of sound these actions involve. There are two possible derivations of this word.

The usual interpretation is:

Hand   Usually read as two moons reflecting each other. (Friend)

This image gives us a good metaphor for the experience of Push Hands, where both people move as if they are each the reflection of the other. But there is another possible source for this character:

Peng may be derived from a primitive character representing the tail of the legendary Chinese Phoenix, the *Fenghuang*. This bird is a symbol of the ying/yang balance and harmony of nature and therefore also of human relations — especially that of marriage.

This primitive character definitely brings to mind the fabulous Chinese Roc, called *Peng*, which appears in Zhuangzi. *Peng* is a monstrous bird representing the power of the air. With its wings like clouds, it can travel tremendous distances with incredible speed. It carries the sky on its back, which is as broad as a mountain. In flight its wings create great spiraling gusts of wind. What a picture to keep in mind as we raise our arms in the *Peng* movement! Either the Phoenix or the Roc is a far cry from the little sparrow, giving a completely different sense of dynamics.

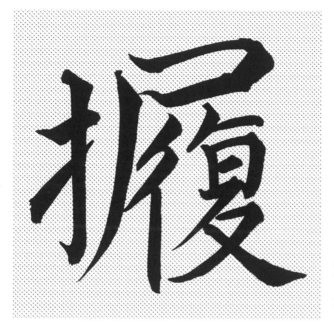

Lu
˅
(lo͝o)

Lu

Lu is an absolutely obscure word – not in any dictionary. But here is a chance to put our game to a test. We look at what is in the character and discover our own meaning. Perhaps it is about the rocking, rolling motion of a boat, and about the balance required to stand in a boat. Or perhaps it is about rowing or poling a boat, where the momentum forward is in unity, harmony, balance and rhythm with the energy exerted backward. Or perhaps you see something else in it.

 Hand

 Modern version of an older character showing the boat shaped straw shoes of ancient China. It is about shoes and walking, and seems to have a connotation of returning.

Boat   Foot   Person

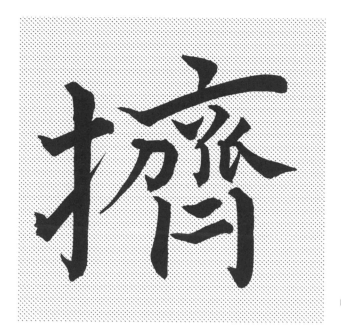

Ji

(jee)

Ji

Pressing, squeezing. Elbowing or shouldering one's way in. The verb used to describe crowding into an elevator or bus . . . Using the hand or arm to join into the whole, to become a part of the harmony or order.

Hand   Modern version of an ancient character showing a cornfield, with the ears at an even height (Harmony, order, a whole)

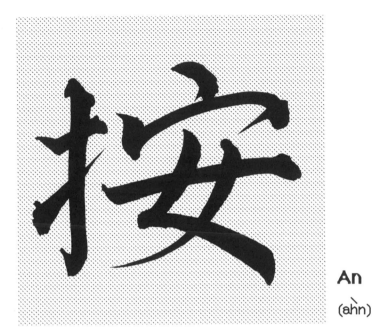

An

(àhn)

An

Examining. Pressing down . . . Placing the hand on. Controlling in harmony with the situation

Hand   Woman under a roof. It is about what the feminine can contribute to a situation. (Peace, tranquility, contentment, intention. Placing or arranging)

This is the verb used for pressing a button or for massage. There is the feeling of connection, and the implication of force used just right.

Peng, Lu, Ji, An are the four basic movements of Taiji, and all of the other movements can be thought of as variations on these themes. These characters all have the hand as the radical – or meaning – element, indicating they have to do with a way of using the hands or arms. Some students of Chinese would say the additional element probably functions only to indicate the pronunciation. But perhaps these pronunciations were chosen because of the associations of the particular word. And perhaps these characters were chosen for the Taiji movements because of those associations. What a happy surprise to find that, although these are the movements fundamental to Taiji as a martial art, the images that make up the characters all have to do with harmony, balance, unity and tranquility!

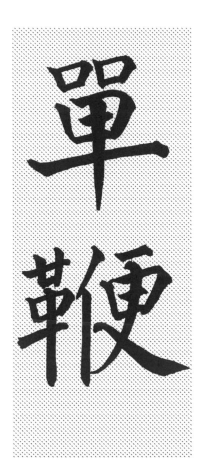

Dan bian

(dahn byan)

Dan

Single . . . Originally, assaulting someone with shouts and a pitchfork, which suggests it may have something to do with piercing sound. How it came to mean single, as opposed to complex, is a mystery to us.

Two mouths representing shouts, cries   Pitchfork

Bian

Whip . . . Leather transforming through its flexibility

Sheepskin spread for drying. (Leather. Wings of a bird. Changing, transforming, removing)

Person changing, improving, acting with ease (The modern dictionary meaning definitely loses something when reduced to (1) convenient, (2) ordinary or (3) to relieve oneself.)

An older version of this character shows:

Fire, bad situation   Armed hand intervening

Here we see both elements of *bian* are about transformation. In the whip images we have a sheepskin in the process of becoming leather and a person who easily improves a situation. The whip's essence is its power to transform, its flexibility, the ease with which it changes shape. And a part of the whip's power is in the singleness, the unity that is transforming. It remains a whip as it is shaped by any force flowing through it. With this in mind, we see the *Dan bian* movement can be about this kind of transformation. The two arms circle together before opening to become one arm, the single whip, deriving its power from the wave-like force of energy flowing through its softness and suppleness.

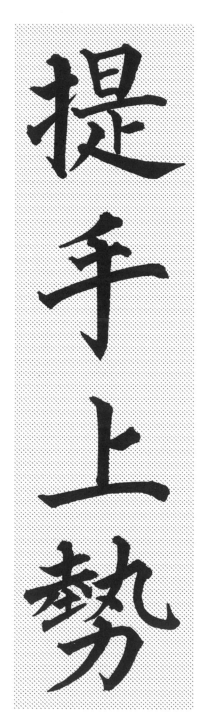

Ti shou shang shi

(tee shoh shahng shuh)

Ti

Lift, raise, put forward . . . Hands or arms moving as the sun moves in its orbit. There is the implication of raising something with weight and substance.

Hand

Order and regularity of the sun's movement, which exemplifies truth according to natural law. (Truth, reality, existence. This, that)

Shou

Hand

This form of hand is a noun, whereas the form in *ti*, above, creates a verb involving the hands or arms.

Shang

Up, higher, first . . . What is above.

Shi

Circumstances. Gesture, aspect . . . Strength required for cultivating the earth.

Sinew, strength

 Cultivating the earth. (Skill, ability. Art, craft)

Earth mound Hand doing something

These characters definitely suggest a feeling of power – of not just raising the arms, but of raising power with the arms.

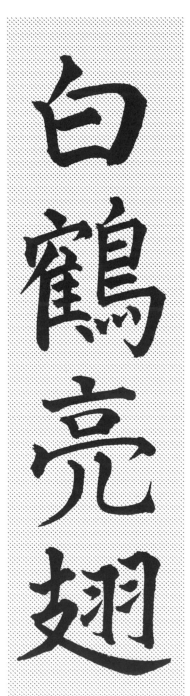

Bai he liang chi
(by huh leeahng ssuh)

Bai

White, pure, clear . . . A ray of light coming from the sun

He

Crane

Bird flying up through space   Bird

Liang

Bright, clear, luminous, shining. Firm. Spreading the wings . . . Superior person.

Raised pavillion. (Height, loftiness)   Person's legs

Chi

Wing . . . The bird's feathered hand opening like a branch.

Hand holding a bough or branch   Pair of wings, feather

The first image of *Bai he liang chi* is the sunbeam of *bai,* which is not only about whiteness, but also carries with it the connotations of enlightenment and transparency. And these are qualities attributed to *he,* the revered white crane of China – the bird able to soar to heaven. It is thought to be a messenger of the gods and a carrier of souls to the next world. This wonderful bird of imposing stature and natural grace is symbolic of purity and nobility.

Furthermore it is graced with a crown of red associated with cinnabar, which represents spiritual illumination. Cinnabar is the *dan* of *dantien,* considered by the Daoist alchemists to be the elixir of life, a spiritual force with many wondrous capacities: to calm the soul, expel evil forces, cure illness, brighten the mind, and heighten the energy. So this spot of red, added to the crane's naturally long life span, insured its place as a symbol of all longevity theories and practices. The white crane can be a metaphor for anyone with lofty aspirations, mundane or other-worldly. In fact one who seeks to attain the Way of Heaven and Earth, the holy person seeking the immortality of oneness in the Dao, is called a *Xianhe* after this bird.

The imagery of the remaining characters, *liang chi,* completes the picture of a marvelous bird standing (perhaps even dancing as cranes do) with spread wings—tall, firm and dazzling in its shining luminosity. Wow! In fact, *liang* is the verb used in Chinese opera for the elegant open-arm stance of the hero identifying himself to the audience after his entrance.

These are associations we can be aware of in our Taiji practice, and each will bring a different quality to our movement. You may have associations coming from your own experience, bringing their own quality to your movement. Trust them and honor them. Find your own way of knowing.

Crane, copy of an old master,
by Margaret Chang (c. 1950)

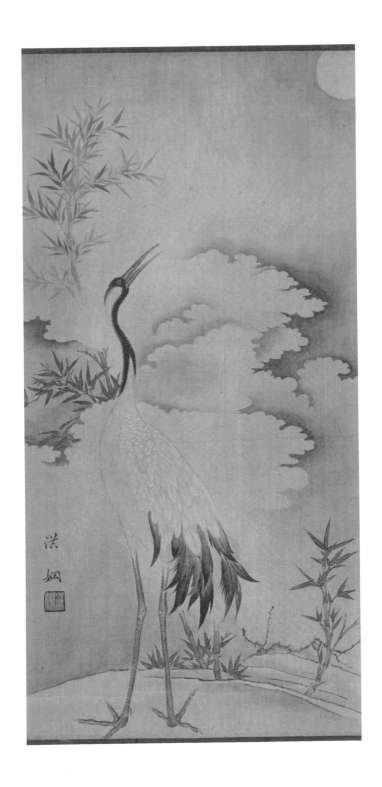

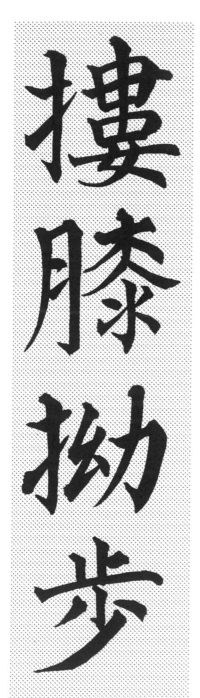

Lou xi ao bu

(lŏh shee aŏh bòo)

Lou

Embracing, hugging, pulling . . . Using the hands and arms to hold a woman.

Hand   Woman held under lock and key for misbehavior. (Trailing along, carrying)

Xi

Knee . . . Tree sap part of the body?

Flesh, parts of the body.   Liquid flowing from a tree. (Sap. Lacquer)

Ao

Pulling, twisting, breaking. Plucking, as a flower . . . Handling silk thread.

Hand   Strength of the thread from silk cocoons. (Tender, slender, young)

Silk Sinew, strength

Bu

Stepping . . . Left and right feet.

The images in *Lou xi ao bu* were at first completely mystifying. But gradually a possible meaning seemed to unfold, a meaning so resonant with my own experience of Taiji, especially of this movement, it has become a favorite.

The images of the first character, *lou,* seem to be about locking up a woman as punishment for her misbehaviour. But in use the word has none of this connotation. It actually has a warm and soft feeling, like a caress, and the dictionary meanings of embracing and hugging reflect this. In fact, *lou* is the verb used for two people dancing together.

Now *xi* is a real puzzle. What does tree sap have to do with the knee? This element of the character may be only a pronunciation indicator, but there is a little nagging hunch of something more there. In fact if we forget the dictionary meaning of knee, and just look at the images, tree sap is a wonderful metaphor for the flowing Taiji energy. Perhaps we can think of *lou xi* as embracing or dancing with the Taiji energy,

This interpretation of the characters somehow seems not quite so far-fetched when we consider along with them the images in *ao.* First we see a hand telling us it is a verb having to do with using the hand or arm. Next to the hand we see a spiraling thread representing a silk cocoon. And next to that is a muscle or sinew signifying strength. Put these all together and we have a picture of the power of movement that is like silk thread in a cocoon – and we are reminded of the Taiji Classics telling us to use energy as if drawing silk from a cocoon.

The silkworm spins its cocoon by spiraling one continuous, delicate thread around itself for protection during its metamophosis from crawling to flying insect. As it is reeled out, the thread unwinds, reversing the way in which it was spun, and spinning the cocoon in turn. This is a powerful metaphor for the quality of Taiji movement and the use of Taiji energy. This silk thread represents the soft flexibility and even continuity of Taiji, as well as the power inherent in a spiral.

Si (Silk) calligraphy, Margaret Chang

The *Lo xi ao bu* movement illustrates this beautifully. The waist turns and the weight shifts, spiraling energy back and in – through the whole body from the soles of the feet. Then the waist turn and weight shift reverse, spiraling energy forward and out – again through the whole body from the soles of the feet, to be delivered by the hands. The dynamics of this spiraling energy is the neutralizing and countering force in Push Hands. There is always a feeling of the flexible spiral of a coiled spring, and this picture of the silk cocoon adds to it even more lightness and mobility.

The imagery here is very simple, but these characters can carry a wonderfully potent picture of dancing with the spiraling Taiji energy.

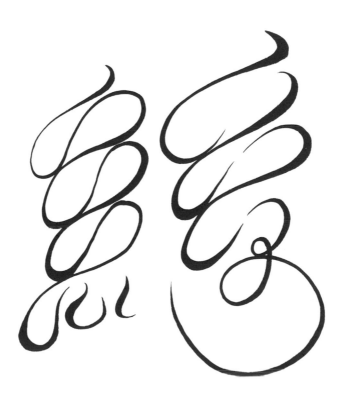

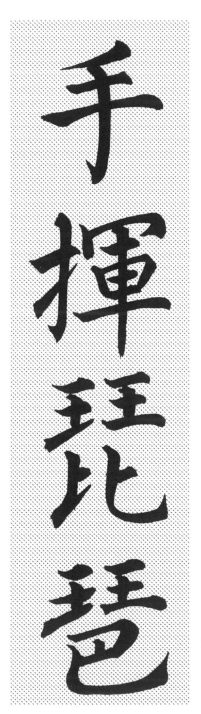

Shou hui pi pa

(shŏh hwāy pée pāh)

Shou Hand

Hui

Wielding, as a sword, conductor's baton or writing brush. Moving, waving, wiping away . . . Commanding an army. There is definitely a connotation of the power and vitality that comes from confidence. You are in command.

Hand   Division of soldiers with chariots. (Army)

Bird's eye view of a carriage showing axle, wheels and cab. (Rolling, revolving, crushing)

Pi Pa The Chinese guitar

Two strings of jade, alluding to the ancient stone chime. This double jade character is used in the names of many other musical instruments.

Uniting with, comparing   Kind of snake, the skin of which is used to cover the pipa.

The pipa, shaped like half of a pear, is held in the arms in front of the body. As with other instruments, its music depends on the hollow space within. Perhaps here it can be considered a metaphor for the whole person of the Taiji artist, suggesting the silent music Taiji can create. You become the pipa.

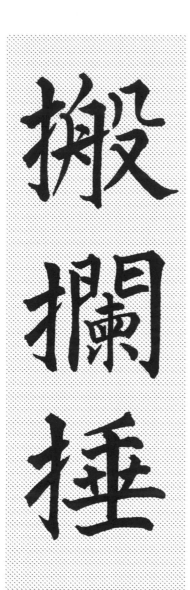

Ban lan chui

(b̄ahn láhn ch́way)

Ban   **Moving, removing, transporting, carrying . . .** Hand circling as if rowing a boat.

Hand

Repeated oar strokes moving a boat. (Manner, sort. Transforming, withdrawing, circling)

Boat   Right hand making a striking motion

Lan   **Hindering, cutting off, blocking . . .** Hand obstructing as if with a door.

Hand   A screened door. (Cutting off, declining. Few, abrupt)

Door   Selecting, choosing.

Chui   **Beating, thumping, pounding . . .** Hand and tree branch. Hitting with a stick or fist.

Hand Tree with foliage. (Hanging, suspending from, dropping down)

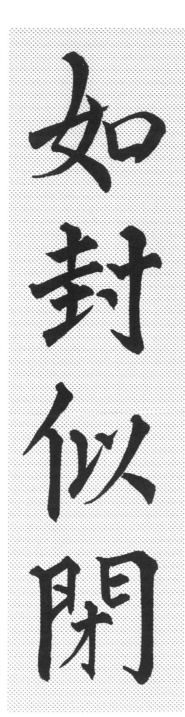

Ru feng si bi

(róo fuhng sùh bèe)

Apparent close 42

Ru

Complying with, according to. As if, like . . .
Speaking in a feminine way. A woman, lacking the physical strength of a man, learns to rely on words and the cunning of complying with a situation to gain advantage.

Woman Mouth

Feng

Protecting territory, sealing up, blockading, closing . . . Measured land, territory.

Tree on a knoll, marking imperial or feudal land

Hand showing the location of the pulse. (The Chinese inch. Measure, authority)

Si

Equal, like, similar. Seem, appear . . . People with the same qualities.

Person Breath or essence of a person. (Virtue, quality)

Bi

Shutting a door. Closing, obstructing . . . Door with a barring device.

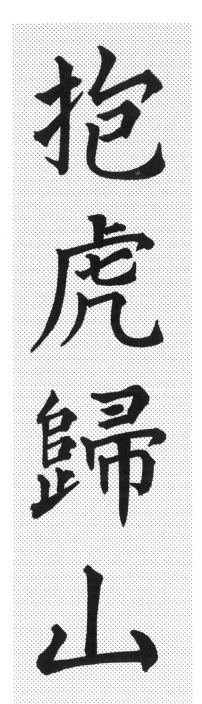

Bao hu gui shan

(baoh hoo gway shahn)

Carry tiger to the mountain   44

Bao Carrying in the arms, holding tight, embracing, cherishing . . . Wrapping up in the arms.

 Hand   Foetus in the womb (Gestation. Wrapping up, containing)

Hu Tiger

 Tiger's stripes   Person's legs

Gui Returning, belonging, restoring, giving back . . Bride (with broom) coming into her husband's family. Woman's marriage

Arriving at a community Broom

Note: In *gui* only a broom represents the bride. At least in *qi*, the actual character for a married woman (shown here), the woman element is included:

Shan Mountain, hill . . . Mountain peaks with valleys between.

Each of the characters of *Bao hu gui shan* is rich in imagery. We begin with *Bao,* which shows a hand and a foetus in the womb. This suggests a special use of the hand, of holding something very precious that offers a promise for a new beginning. And then we learn that what we are holding in this way is Tiger, of all things!

Tiger is one of those beings resonating with the human spirit in such a way that it carries with it a tremendous wealth of ambivalent symbol and metaphor. It can represent danger and the power of darkness, but at the same time can be a protector against evil. In either capacity it stands for authority, courage and ferocity, and it is always a symbol of power and energy. For our purposes here we are considering Tiger as a symbol of the Taiji yin/yang energy, because its very essence is the unity of great power and strength with feline softness and grace.

The imagery of *gui* could be read as the return of the borrowed broom. But we will choose to overlook the implications here and focus on the idea of marriage – another instance of yin/yang unity – as a return to a place of belonging as well as a beginning.

And this place of belonging and beginning is Mountain – symbol of the Sacred Center, of stillness and paradise – yet another image of yin/yang wholeness. It is where heaven and earth come together in a pivot point of equilibrium.

So, read this way, *Bao hu gui shan* could be about embracing the Taiji energy, perhaps even as a foetus in the womb, and returning to the stillness of the center, or the stillness of before the beginning. We keep returning to this movement at the end of each section of the form. In the end is the beginning.

Hu calligraphy, Liu Yung-Fu (18thcentury)
Courtesy, Tseng Yu-Ho

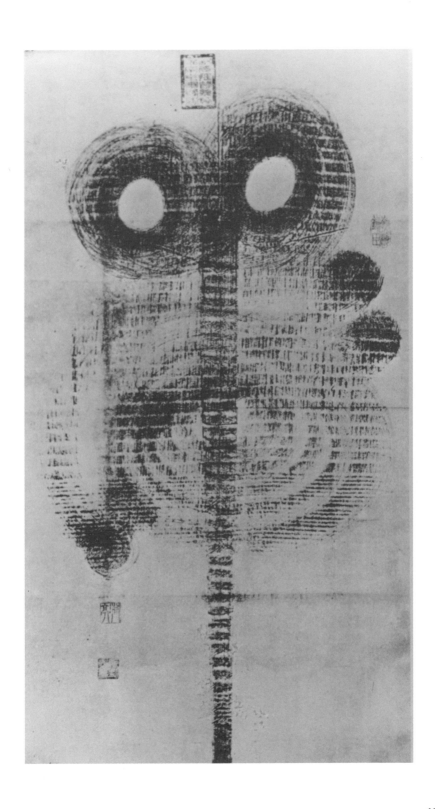

Carry tiger to the mountain   47

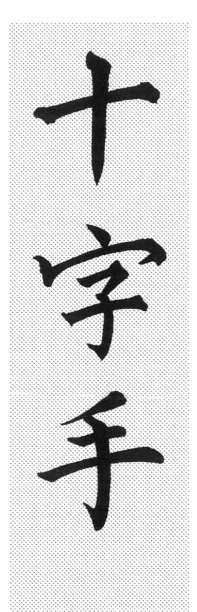

Shi zi shou
(shúh zùh shŏh)

Shi Zi **The Cross, crossroads** . . . Where the apparent opposites converge to create the center.

Ten. The number containing all other numbers. Completion. Symbol of extension – the four cardinal points and the center.

Baby under a roof. Bearing and nursing children Chinese characters, which were born of the combination of ancient primitive picture-words

Shou Hand

Shi zi means the character for ten, which takes the form of the cross, yet another symbol of the yin/yang unity of heaven and earth. But this time there is an emphasis on the center, where all comes together in wholeness and completeness.

The *Shi zi shou* movement also represents a completion, both in the sense of an ending and a wholeness. In the Taiji form we have been involved in the extension of our body and our energy in all directions. But here we bring everything together into the center. This is what we do on the mountaintop. We bring the tiger energy in to our center. Now we are in a position for either an ending or a new beginning.

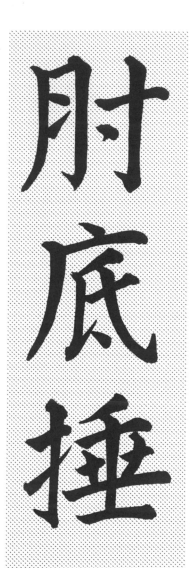

Zhou di chui

(joh dee chway)

Zhou Forearm. Elbow . . . Part of the arm above the wrist.

Flesh, parts of the body   Hand showing the pulse at the wrist. (The Chinese inch)

Di **Base, foundation, end. Underneath, below . . .** What is at the bottom of something. The heart of the matter.

Half of a hut. (Shed, shop)

Floating plant, which has put its roots down in the bottom of a pond. (Bottom, foundation. Sinking)

Chui **Beating, thumping, pounding . . .** Hand and tree branch. Hitting with a stick or fist.

Hand   Tree with foliage. (Hanging, suspending from, dropping down)

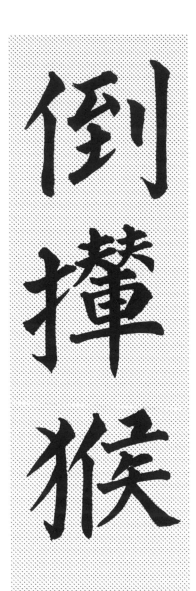

Dao nian hou

(dàoh nyǎhn hóh)

Dao

Upside down, inverted or in reverse . . . The images are simply of a person arriving. There is no suggestion of arriving in any of these strange ways.

Person   Arriving at a destination (Reaching, going to)

Bird, with spread wings, landing on earth

Knife, sword

Nian

Ousting, driving away, catching up . . . Driving with the hand.

Hand   Men pulling a carriage. (Transporting)

Men   Wheeled vehicle, carriage

Hou

Monkey. Clever child . . . Beautiful, aristocratic animal. What else but the monkey?

Dog, animal

Person standing beside a target pierced by an arrow. (Skill in archery, virtue. Aristocrat. Beautiful, excellent)

Monkey is important in Chinese myth, both as one of the animals of the zodiac and as the outrageous hero of the Chinese classic, *Journey to the West,* where he represents human intellect. As such, his adventures are sometimes wonderful and sometimes terrible – but always lively and hilarious. However, when we consider both the name and the movement of *Dao nian hou,* the story that comes to mind is one told by Zhuangzi:

> Once, when the Duke of Wu went to hunt on Monkey Mountain, the terrified monkeys, as usual, ran away to hide in the treetops as soon as they saw him. But there was one monkey who used the opportunity of this audience to show off his great agility by swinging from branch to branch through the trees. When the Duke shot at it, the monkey caught the flying arrow in its hand! Then the Duke ordered his men to shoot and soon the monkey fell dead, pierced by many arrows. The Duke said to his companion, Yen Pui, "Do you see what happened to this animal when it flaunted its skill and cleverness? Remember to not rely on distinction and talent in your dealings with people." Returning home, Yen Pui got rid of all that made him stand out from others, and as a result was held in awe by everyone.

Perhaps this story is what the Taiji movement is about. We learn to step back, and to get rid of the monkey quality of wanting to stand out – of seeking distinction. Laozi also has something to say about this, as in chapter seven, where the Sage finds himself ahead when he places himself behind. He finds self-realization and self-preservation in self-forgetting.

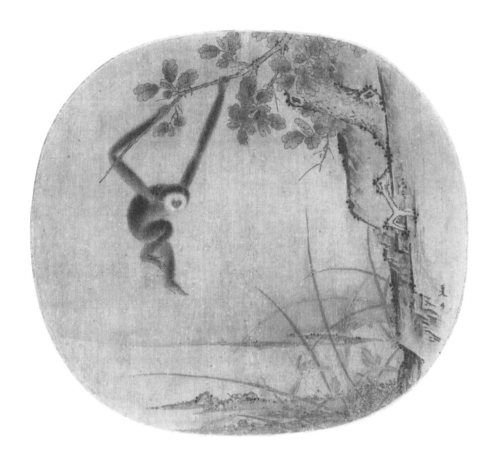

Swinging Gibbon attributed to Hsia Kuei (c. 1180-1224)
Southern Song dynasty. Fan mounted as album leaf, 24.8 x 34.8 cm.
© The Cleveland Museum of Art, 1996, John L. Severance Fund, 1978.1

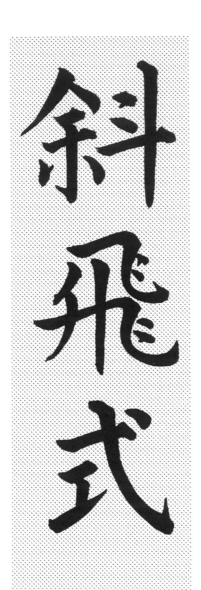

Xie fei shi

(shyeh fay shuh)

Xie

Inclining, tilting, oblique, slanting . . . Measuring a roof.

Thatched roof. Its meaning of I, me, comes from the custom of calling out one's name and purpose when entering a home.

Ten ladles. (A peck)

Fei

Flying, hovering, soaring. Quick, high . . . Crane flying with fluttering wings.

Shi

Style, form, ritual, mood, posture . . . Work following a pattern. Imitating.

Carpenter's square. (Labor, skill, work)

Hook, arrow, pin, tool for pointing or marking

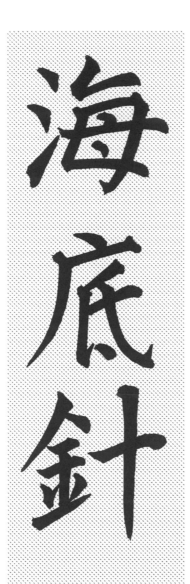

Hai di zhen

(h̆y děe ju̅hn)

Hai

Sea, ocean . . . Mother of waters and of all life.

Water

Woman with breasts, mother. Above her is vegetation, life. Perhaps the mother of all life (Each, every)

Di

Base, foundation, end. Underneath, below . . . What is at the bottom of something. The heart of the matter.

Half of a hut (Shed, shop)

Floating plant, which has put its roots down in the bottom of a pond. (Bottom, foundation. Sinking)

Zhen

Needle, pin, sting, probe, stitch . . . Sharp, pointed, metallic object.

Mineral, metal, gold

 Pointed, piercing object

Needle at the bottom of the sea   59

On hearing "needle at the bottom of the sea," two stories come to mind. The first is another story about Monkey, from Wu Chengen's *Journey to the West*:

> Once upon a time Monkey was on a quest for the perfect weapon. His search led him to the bottom of the Eastern Sea, where he was received by the Dragon King. There all the weapons he tried out were either too light or too heavy, until the Dragon Mother gave him the holy iron rod which had been used to pound the Milky Way flat. Monkey found this to be the perfect weapon because he could use his magic powers to shrink it from its twenty foot length to two feet for fighting, and then to the size of a needle to stick behind his ear.

The other story we are reminded of is:

> There was once an old Daoist monk who was known for his skill at embroidering. People who came to admire his work would often ask him to teach them the secret of his ability to create such beauty. He always told them, "I can only show you what my hands do. I can not show you the Golden Needle that produces them. You must find that for yourself."

The Golden Needle is found at the bottom of the sea – in the deep reservoir that is the source of all creativity.

Priest Sewing Under the Morning Sun
Kao (c.1350) Nambokucho period, Japan.
Hanging scroll, ink on paper, 83.7 x 34.8 cm.
© The Cleveland Museum of Art, 1996,
John L. Severance fund, 1962.163

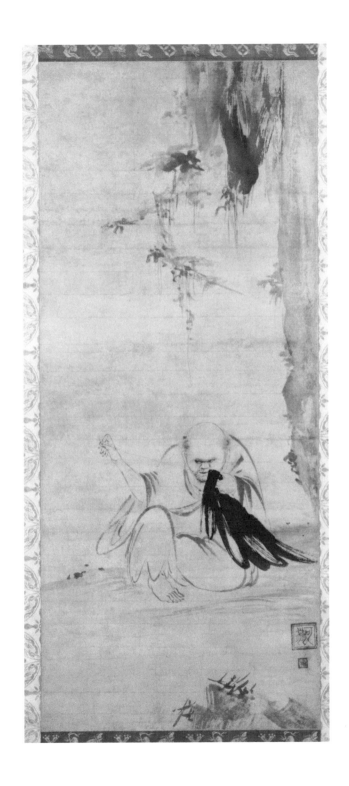

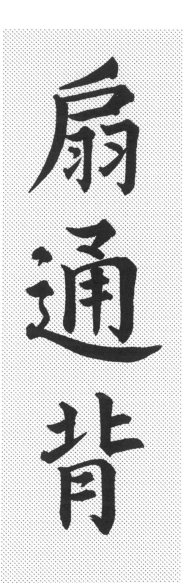

Shan tong bei

(shahn tong bay)

Fan through the back 62

Shan   **Fanning, inciting, instigating . . .** Opening and closing movement of wings or doors.

 Door   Pair of wings. Feather

Tong   **Opening, clearing out, understanding, connecting . . .** Movement of an inner force allowing the bud to open into a flower.

Moving, flowing   Opening of a flower bud in a sacred vessel. (Blooming. Path)

Bei   **Back, behind . . .** Part of the body presented in disagreement or defeat.

Two persons turned away from each other (Disagreeing, defeating. North)

Flesh, parts of the body

The characters *Shan tong bei* give us beautiful imagery for the internal feeling of Taiji energy we can experience as we move. The doors and wings of *shan* suggest the wave-like rhythm of the flow of energy we feel in *tong,* in the sacred vessel of the body, as it rises through *bei,* the back, the spine, to open above like a big flower or fan. And in doing the movement, the whole body seems to describe this experience. Together, the elements of the character *tong* create a picture that is especially expressive of the openess, clarity, continuity and flow of Taiji movement and energy.

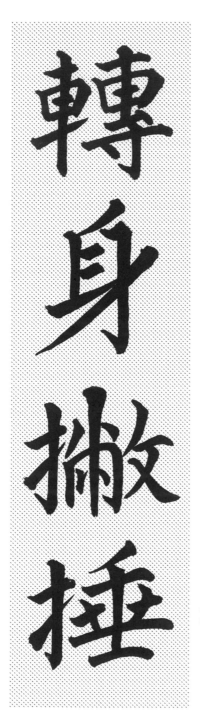

Zhuan shen pie chui

(jooan shuhn pyeh chway)

Turn and chop with fist　　**64**

Zhuan

Turning around, revolving, rotating, changing ... Special, defining characteristic of a wheel.

Wheeled vehicle. Machine. (Rolling, revolving, crushing)

Small notebook worn on the wrist. (Only, special)

Shen

Body, person, oneself, life duration ... Person with a big belly. The primitive meaning was conception.

Pie

Throwing away, rejecting, abandoning. A brushstroke down ... Motion of hand tearing

Hand   Piece of cloth with holes. (Rag, tatters)

Hand tearing the cloth

Chui

Beating, thumping, pounding ... Hand and tree branch. Hitting with a stick or fist.

Hand   Tree with foliage. (Hanging, suspending from, dropping down)

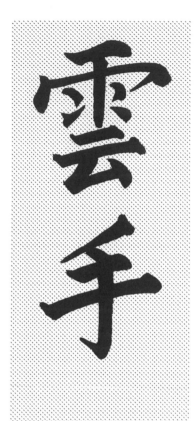

Yun shou

(yóon shǒh)

Yun

Clouds, cloudy. Gathering . . . Vapors rising to heaven to condense and return to earth as rain.

Cloud hanging from heaven with falling drops of water. (Rain)

Vapors rising up to heaven. (Cloud. Speaking)

Shou   Hand

Clouds represent the transforming, changing patterns of things. The essence of clouds is their constantly changing form as they are created, carried and shaped by the forces of nature. They are soft and floating, but within their insubstantiality there is the potential for thunder and lightning and the force of storms.

Then, when we look at the images in *yun*, we become aware of the cloud as a part of the whole yin/yang process of the rain cycle. We see vapor rising in response to the light of heaven, gathering into cloud and transforming into rain, which falls in response to earth's gravity only to be transformed again into vapor.

These cloud images are all important to the quality of our Taiji movement. Are our cloud hands soft and insubstantial enough to to go along with any changing circumstance? Are they at the same time capable of strength and power? Are they circling – rising and falling in response to the energies of heaven and earth? And are they moving with the soft beauty of clouds?

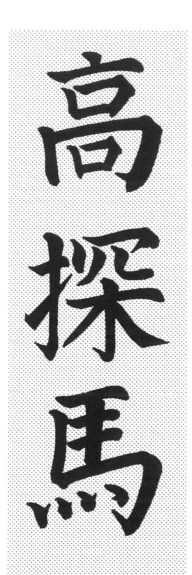

Gao tan ma

(gaoh tahn mǎh)

Gao

High, exalted, tall, noble. Skill . . . Pavillion built on top of another structure. An elevated place.

Tan

Exploring, seeking, visiting, trying, testing, going deep . . . This is the verb used for a detective's searching for evidence or a suspect. Reaching into the depths of the fireplace.

Hand

The space in the Chinese stove for burning wood (Deep, profound)

Hole made by removing earth, cave

 Tree, wood

Ma

Horse. At once, immediately, rapidly. Power, perseverance . . . Horse, with mane and tail flying.

Tan Ma is used for a scout, or scouting.

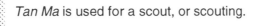

These wonderful images of *Gao tan ma* might suggest climbing up onto a horse in order to search for something. Or they might suggest the testing of your personal horsepower – the heights and depths of it. Is your horse in good shape?

They also might bring to mind Zhuangzi's parable about horses:

Horses have hooves that carry them over frost and snow, and they have hair that protects them from wind and cold. They eat grass and drink water, and prance with tails held high. This is the true nature of horses. They have no use for fine halls and great dwellings.

But one day Bo Le, the famous horse trainer, came along saying, "I am good at managing horses." And since then things have never been the same for horses. He branded them, clipped their hair and pared their hooves. He put halters and bridles on them. He hobbled them and put them in stables. As a result two or three of every ten died. Then he kept them hungry and thirsty, and taught them to trot and gallop in formation, using a bit in front and a whip behind. Because of this good management more than half of them died.

With this story in mind, perhaps we can think of *Gao tan ma* as a testing of the quality of our movement. Are we able to move with the kind of integrity, simplicity and clarity of natural, organic movement the horses had before the trainer/manager took over? For most of us, the practice of Taiji is actually a process of unlearning – a letting go of all the harnesses and trappings we seem to acquire along the way – a searching for our own natural integrity.

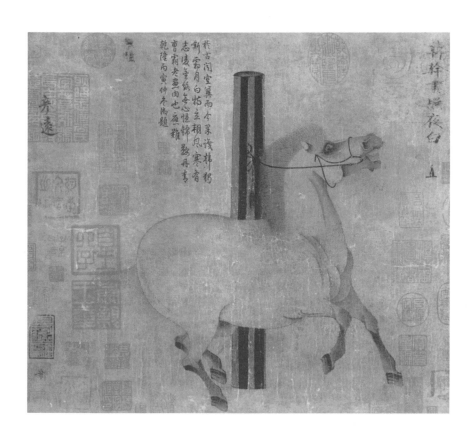

Night-Shining White Han Kan (8th century).
Tang dynasty. Ink on paper, 30 x 30.8 cm.
The Metropolitan Museum of Art,
The Dillon Fund, 1977. (1977.78)

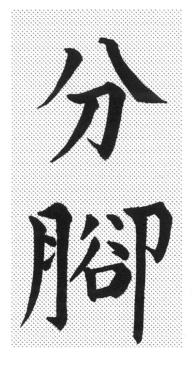

Fen jiao

(fuhn jyǎoh)

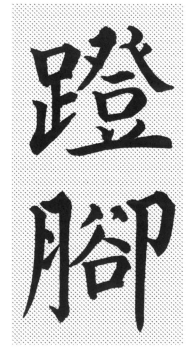

Deng jiao

(duhng jyǎoh)

Fen

Dividing, separating, parting, distinguishing . .
Something cut with a knife.

Separation, division   Knife

Jiao

Foot, leg, base . . . Since the images here seem to have something to do with a stiff upper lip, we have to concede that here, while the flesh element pertains to the meaning, the other elements only indicate the pronunciation.

Flesh, parts of the body   Flesh above the mouth. (Upper lip)

 Scepter. (Authority, rule. Restraining)

Deng

Climbing, stepping on, treading . . . This is the verb used for going up a mountain, a ladder or stairs.

Foot   Ascending, going up.

Feet, moving one at a time Raised platform

Jiao

Foot, leg, base. This is the same *jiao* as above.

These two ways of using the feet or legs can be related to the horseride of the previous movement. We have to open to allow for the space of the horse beneath us, and we have to climb up onto the horse to ride it.

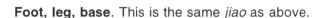

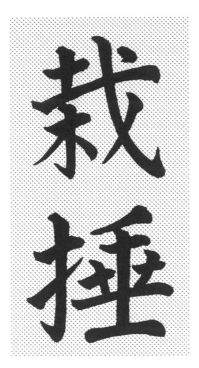

Zai chui

(z̄y chẃay)

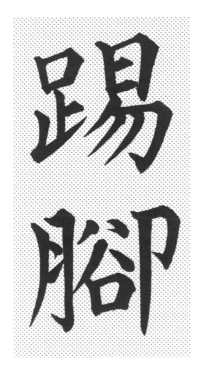

Ti jiao

(t̄ee jyǎoh)

Zai Planting, inserting, falling, imposing something on someone.

Weapon or tool thrust into the earth, out of which emerges a plant (Wounding)   Tree

Chui Beating, thumping, pounding . . . Hand and tree branch. Hitting with a stick or fist.

Hand Tree with foliage. (Hanging, suspending from, dropping down)

This is another instance where knowledge of the Chinese word can change the whole quality of the Taiji movement.

Ti Kicking . . . The verb used for football and soccer. Easy, changing foot.

Foot Lizard, chameleon. (Changing, transforming. Easy, alert. The *Yi* of *Yijing*)

Jiao Foot, leg, base. Since the images here seem to have something to do with a stiff upper lip, we have to concede that here, while the flesh element pertains to the meaning, the other elements only indicate the pronunciation.

Flesh, parts of the body Flesh above the mouth. (Upper lip)

Scepter. (Authority, rule. Restraining)

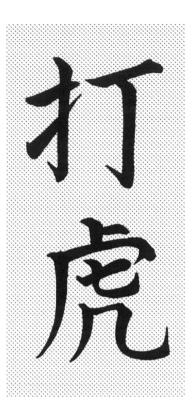

Da hu

(dǎh hǒo)

Da

Among the many meanings of this character are striking, hitting, breaking, fighting, building, stirring, drawing, painting, spreading, opening, sending, gathering, reaping, receiving, catching, hunting, estimating, doing, playing and using. It is the verb used for Taiji, for ball games, for meditation and for whispering, as well as for flogging, threshing, destroying, ramming, robbing, spanking, smashing, sweeping, typing, forging iron, etc . . . Hand with a nail. The movement of driving a nail. It's pretty wild to consider how these many possible meanings could be used with the . . . . .

Hu

Tiger

Tiger's stripes   Person's legs

If we are thinking of Tiger as a metaphor for our Taiji energy, what a multitude of uses for it are presented to us by the word *da*! But we can also think of Tiger as symbolic of the situations we deal with in life, and Zhuangzi has a Tiger tale that is pertinent here:

When Yan He was appointed tutor to the crown prince, son of the Duke of Wei, he sought advice from Ju Boyu, a minister of the state. "The prince is a cruel man, depraved and murderous. If I let him follow his violent nature the country may be endangered. If I try to curb it, I may be endangered. He is able to see the faults of others, but he cannot see his own faults. How shall I deal with a man like this?"

"Good question!" said Ju Boyu. "Be cautious and aware. You must not try to improve him but to improve yourself. Be flexible and in tune with him, but keep your own center. Follow him but do not allow yourself to be pulled off balance or you will be overthrown and destroyed. Harmonize with him but do not be pulled into his evil ways or you will be criticized and condemned. If he wants to be childish, erratic or reckless, be childish, erratic or reckless with him. Know his nature, and you can lead him to where you want him to be.

Then Ju Boyu went on to say: "You need to know how the tiger trainer accomplishes his job. He never gives the tiger a live animal to eat so it will not develop its instinct for killing. He never even gives it a whole dead animal to eat so it will not it develop its instinct for tearing apart. He is constantly aware of the tiger's appetite and sensitive to its ferocious nature. Though tigers are very different from men, they can be controlled and trained to be gentle by understanding tiger nature and going along with it. Only those who go against it are harmed."

This advice sounds very familiar to Taiji artists! Here Zhuangzi gives us the ideas at the root of Taiji as a way of self-defense, which can be projected into a way of living. It is a way of handling situations with no aggression, violence, or opposition. It is a way of overcoming by yielding.

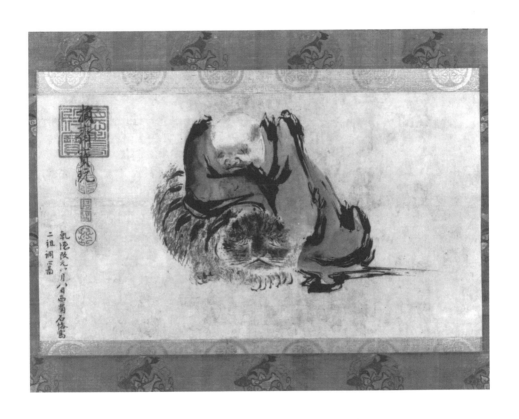

The Second Patriarch in Contemplation, attributed to Shi Ke
Southern Song dynasty (13th cent.) 47 x 36.5 cm
Collection of The Tokyo National Museum

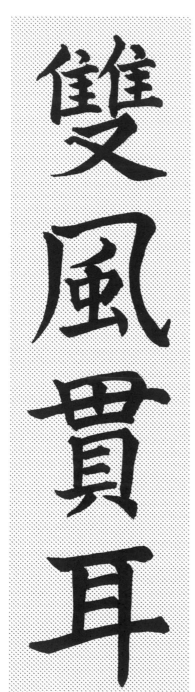

Shuang feng guan er

(shwahng fuhng gwahn ar)

Shuang Pair, two, double, both . . . Two birds in one hand.

Two birds   Hand

Feng Wind, breath, abuse, style, scene . . . Motion and extension. Crawling everywhere across the earth.

The one in all. Unity in diversity. (All, generally, every, ordinary)

Crawling animals. Snakes, worms, insects

Guan Piercing, passing through, stringing, tying, linking together . . . Cowry shells strung together.

Two objects strung together. (Piercing, stringing)

Cowry shell, used in ancient China as money

Er Ear

Two winds rushing through the ears to pierce the head – a pain filled image for a self defense movement or a metaphor for what?

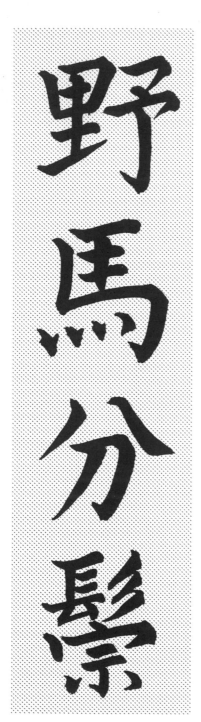

Ye ma fen zong
˘ ˘ ‒ ‒
(yeh mah fuhn zong)

Ye

Wild, uncultivated. Untamed, rustic, unruly . . .
Frontier farming communities who dealt with the barbarian tribes of the open country.

Cultivated field. (Inside, inner. Neighborhood, hometown. Mile)

Hands giving and receiving. (Communicating, connecting. Me, I)

Ma

Horse. At once, immediately, rapidly. Power, perseverance . . . Horse, with mane and tail flying.

In addition to being the unspoiled horse in the Zhuangzi story told on page 70, *ye ma* is also used for dust clouds and mirages.

Fen

Dividing, separating, parting, distinguishing . .
Something cut with a knife.

Separation, division   Knife

Zong

Horse's mane . . . Perhaps the most distinguished long hair.

Long hair held by a pin. (Long, growing)   Hair, feathers

Building associated with heaven or the divine. (Ancestral temple. Ancestors, clan, kind, kindred, sect. The most distinguished. Following)

The Zhuangzi story on page 70 tells of Bo Le destroying the true nature and integrity of wild horses by training them. The wild horse appears two more times in Zhuanzi, where it is a metaphor for the heart/mind. The Chinese have one word for both heart and mind, clearly showing a very basic difference from our way of thinking.

These two stories from Zhuanzi are:

Cui Ju asked Laozi, "If all under heaven is not governed, how will the human heart/mind be made good?" To this Laozi replied, "You must very carefully never interfere with it. If you try to force it down, it will only spring back higher. It can be gentle and soft or sharp and hard. It can be fiery and hot or icy and cold. In a wink it can go twice beyond the four seas and back again. Resting, it is still as a deep pool. Moving, it can reach to heaven. The heart/mind is a wild horse that can not be tied down."

And:

The Daoist monk, Yancheng Ziyou, once said to his teacher, Dongguo Ziqi: "As I studied Dao, in the first year I was like a wild horse, in the second year I became gentle, in the third year I became free from cares, in the fourth year I became one with all things, in the fifth year the many became one, in the sixth year I became filled with spirit, in the seventh year I followed my original nature, in the eighth year life and death lost their meaning for me, and in the ninth year I attained the Great Mystery."

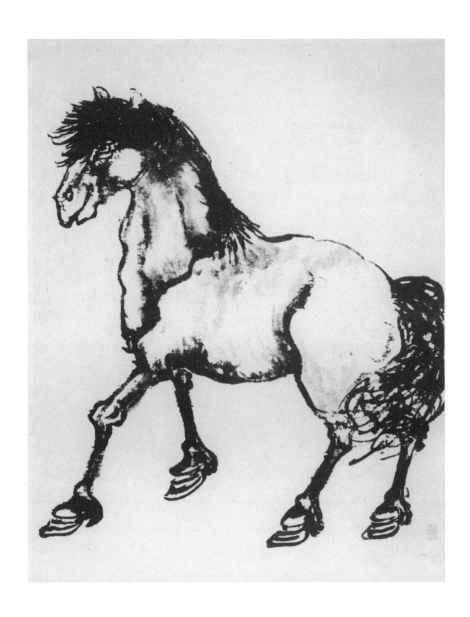

Horse, Jin Nong (18th century)
Collection unknown.

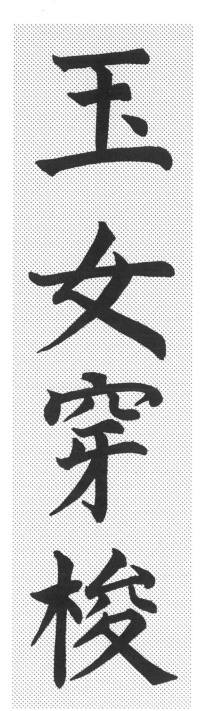

Yu nu chuan suo
ˋ　ˇ　－　－
(yoo noo chwahn swoh)

Fair lady works at shuttle　**86**

Yu

Gem, jade, valuable. Pure, fair, beautiful . . .
Pieces of jade strung together

Nu

女

Woman, girl, female

Chuan

穿

Penetrating, passing through, crossing. Wearing, putting on . . . Biting through

Hole made by removing earth. Cave Teeth

Suo

Weaver's shuttle. Moving back and forth . . .
Walking wood

Tree, wood Person walking slowly and solemnly

In many mythologies weaving represents the fabric of the universe, suggesting a kind of cosmic loom. It is a wonderful image of the mutual dependency of the two primal forces. What is unusual here is that we seem to have the feminine as the active force – the yang within the yin. The beautiful woman weaves a wholeness of yin weft and yang warp, providing the substance necessary for creation.

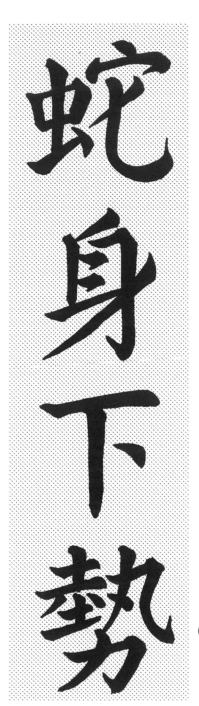

She shen xia shi

(shúh shuhn shyàh shùh)

Snake creeps down   **88**

She

Snake, serpent. At ease, contented (when pronounced differently)

Crawling animal

Coiled snake, with its tongue sticking out. (Easy, at ease, loose. That, he, she, it)

Shen

Body, person, oneself, life duration . . . Person with a big belly. The primitive meaning was conception.

Xia

Below, down, under. Descending, using, capturing, yielding, finishing, taking away

Shi

Circumstances. Gesture, aspect . . . Strength required for cultivating the earth.

Sinew, strength   Cultivating the earth. (Skill, ability. Art, craft)

Earth mound   丸 Hand doing something

Snake is so rich in associations we will consider only a few that might pertain to its use in the names of Taiji movements. It's flexibility combined with strength make it another symbol of the yin/yang Taiji energy. It represents the spine and the energy of the spinal chord. It is considered to be the possessor of secret knowledge. And because of its ability to shed its skin, it is also symbolic of transformation and rebirth.

Legend has it that a fight between a crane and a snake was the original inspiration for Taiji. The crane uses its powerful wings to defend itself – opening and closing, raising and lowering them. The snake's defense is its sinuous curling and straightening, as well as its calm awareness. It can easily recoil from a strike, simultaneously yielding and firm. The essence of both crane and snake is found in Taiji movement. And the essence of both is found in the flying serpent, the dragon, with its remarkable ability to appear or disappear – always at the appropriate time.

Maybe Zhuangzi's tale about Shade and Shadow belongs here:

> Shade once said to Shadow, "Sometimes you move, sometimes you are still. Sometimes you sit down, sometimes you stand up. Why are you so capricious?" Shadow answered, "Perhaps my actions are in accord with Something Else, and perhaps that Something Else also acts in accord with another Something Else. Perhaps my movement is like that of a snake's scales or of a cicada's wings. How can I tell why I do one thing and not another?"

This story can be interpreted in many ways and on many levels. It can illustrate the quality of Push Hands, where we learn to flow with our partner's movement without resisting and without letting go – as a shadow, or as the skin of a snake or the wings of a cicada. It can also be a good illustration of a greater lesson we might learn. That is the possibility of extending this same quality in order to live our lives in harmony, unity, balance and rhythm with whatever comes our way, and ultimately with all that is and is not.

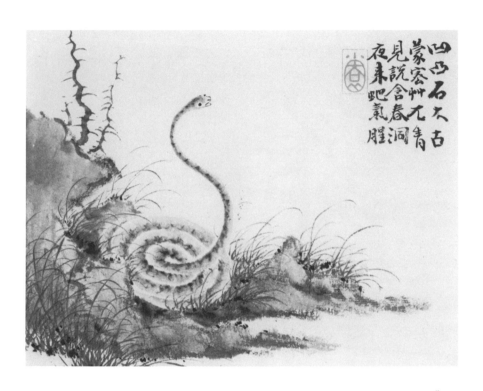

四山凹凸石太古
蒙茸艸木青
見說含春洞
夜來虵氣腥

Snake, Xin Luo (1684-1761)
Album leaf: Ink on paper
P.S. Lim Collection

Snake creeps down 91

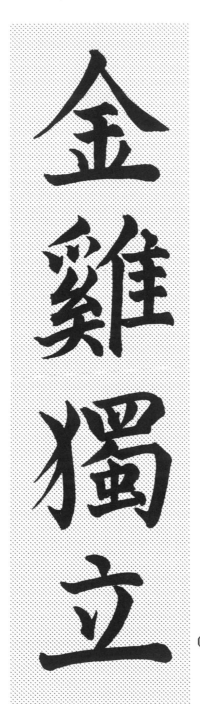

Jin ji du li

(jin jee dóo lèe)

Golden pheasant stands on one leg

Jin

Metal, gold, golden . . . Mineral deposits in the earth's strata. Crystalline, inorganic matter

Ji

Chicken, fowl, young bird, child. The _jin ji_ is the golden pheasant of China . . . Bird working with silk thread?

Hand working with silk thread. (The interrogative. What, how, why, where)

 Bird

Du

Only, single, alone . . . Silkworm spinning a cocoon around itself

Dog, animal

Head of a silkworm and the movement of its body

 Crawling animals

Li

Stand, set up, exist. Immediate . . . Person standing on the earth. _Du li_ means standing alone, independent.

Again we have some marvelous images to play with. We begin with *jin ji,* the golden bird. This could be interpreted in may ways – usually as the radiant cock, the yang bird of dawn. But it could be the golden pheasant, which is called *jin ji,* and is the bird frequently used for illustrating the mythological Phoenix, the *Fenghuang,* mentioned in our notes on *Peng* (p.19). Both of these birds symbolize light, virtue, and prosperity. So take your pick. What the images tell us here is that it is a golden bird that handles silk thread, and of course that doesn't make any sense. The silk handling element is probably just a phonetic.

But when we look at the images of *du,* we find another silk image – the image of a silkworm spinning its cocoon. This doesn't make any sense either, until we realize how beautifully it expresses the meaning of only, single and alone. The silk thread spiraling around the worm establishes its "onliness" and its "all oneness." The silkworm is contained and protected at the center of the cocoon during its transformation into a winged creature. This picture of the silkworm spinning its cocoon could be a metaphor for Taiji. As we move through the form, we draw around ourselves continuous circular patterns of energy, in which we find centeredness, oneness, containment and protection.

When we add *li,* we have *du li* – standing alone – and we are reminded of another Zhuangzi story:

> Once King Huan gave Ji Xingzi a fine fighting cock to train. At the end of ten days, the king asked, "Is it time for me to organize a tournament?" "Definitely not," the trainer replied. "This cock is too vain – too anxious to show off its strength and fighting skills."

> At the end of another ten days, the king asked again, "Now is it time to organize a cockfight?" And Ji Xingzi replied, "No, not yet. This bird still has much anger. Its spirit is still too belligerent when it hears another cock crow, even in the next village."

But finally, at the end of yet another ten days, Ji Xingzi said, "At last it is a true fighting cock. Now when it hears another cock crow, it stands like a wooden cock. It stands completely immobile, in calm serenity. Its virtue is whole. Now no other bird will brave a fight with it but will quickly run away."

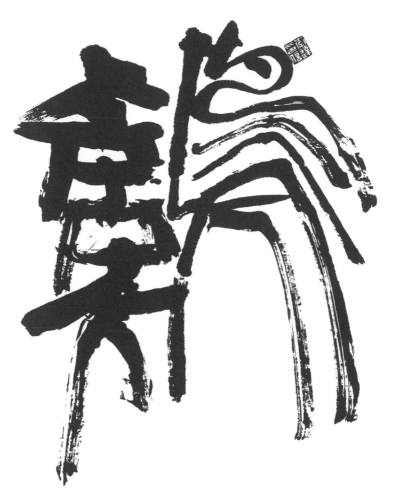

Ji calligraphy, Li Lida (1922-1982)
Courtesy, Li Ai-Ling

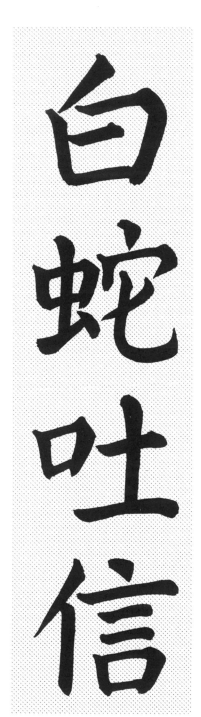

Bai she tu xin

(bý shúh too shìn)

White snake sticks out its tongue   96

Bai

White, pure, clear . . . A ray of light coming from the sun

She

Snake, serpent. Or it can mean: at ease, contented (when pronounced differently)

Crawling animal

Coiled snake, with its tongue sticking out. (Easy, at ease, loose. That, he,she,it)

Tu

Spitting, vomiting, disclosing, giving up unwillingly . . . Mouth and soil

Mouth   Earth, soil

Xin

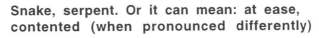

Truth, sincerity, faith. Believing, trusting. Mail, letter, message, information. Freely, easily, aimlessly . . . Person standing behind his word

Person Sound coming from the mouth. (Words. Speaking, telling)

In China *she tu xin* is used for the snake sticking out its tongue, but we think it could just as well be about the white snake revealing the truth, or disclosing its secret knowledge.

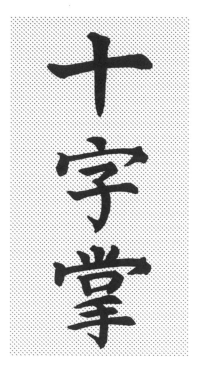

Shi zi zhang

(shúh zùh jaȟng)

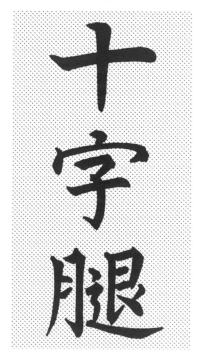

Shi zi tui

(shúh zùh twǎy)

Shi Zi

The Cross, crossroads . . . Where the apparent opposites converge to create the center.

Ten. The number containing all other numbers. Completion. Symbol of extension – the four cardinal points and the center

Baby under a roof. Bearing and nursing children. (Chinese characters, which were born of the combination of ancient primitive picture-words)

Zhang

The palm. Holding in the hand, wielding, controlling . . . Main part of the hand

Chinese house showing the crest of the roof, the finishing touch. (Superior) Hand

Shi Zi

The Cross, crossroads . . . This is the same *shi zi* as above.

Tui

Leg . . . Part of the body for walking

Flesh, parts of the body Person moving along, walking

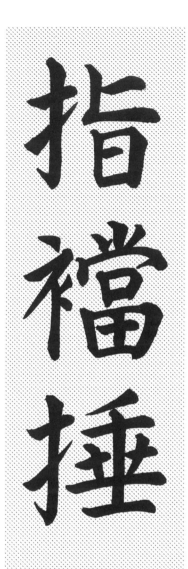

Zhi dang chui

(juh dahng chway)

Zhi

Finger. Pointing, directing . . . Part of the hand used for indicating

Hand   Modern version of this ancient character showing the tongue tasting something sweet (Good, excellent. An imperial decree. Intending, meaning)

Dang

Trousers, crotch or seat of trousers . . . valuable part of clothing?

Garment, clothes

Value of a field or house. (Equaling, matching, compensating. Convenient)

Chinese house with roof crest   Field

Chui

Beating, thumping, pounding . . . Hand and tree branch. Hitting with a stick or fist

Hand   Tree with foliage. (Hanging, suspending from, dropping down)

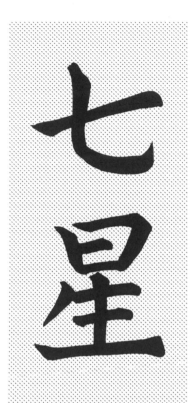

Qi xing

(chee shing)

Qi   Seven

Xing   **Star** . . . Living sun. Giving birth to light.

Sun, light   Growing plant (Giving birth to, living)

Weiger says the ancient character shows "the quintessence of sublimated matter, that ascended and crystallized into stars."

Here, in our Taiji movement, our forearms seem to form the character *qi* as they cross in front of our face. We can think of this as a sort of salute to the seven stars of the Northern Dipper, considered in China to be the sacred, polar center of cosmic order. It is called the Heavenly Gates, and it represents the place of origin and return, the unmoved mover, and the still point of the turning heavens. To reach the seven stars is to be in unity, rhythm and harmony with the movement of the universe.

What a delightful surprise it was to discover that The Northern Dipper plays a great part in some ancient Daoist meditations. One of these is a moving meditation called Pacing the Dipper, or Pacing the Network of Heaven. Evidently this constellation, along with the network of stars surrounding it, is drawn on the earth as a kind of labyrinth. The meditator then dances along this in a prescribed way – finally reaching the last star (which is the Celestial Gate), turns, and "is elevated to the higher realms of heaven."

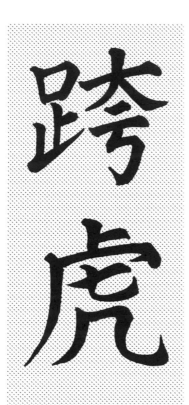

Kua hu

(kẁah hŏo)

Kua

Stepping, striding, straddling, going beyond, excelling . . . Using the feet in an exaggerated or showy way?

Foot

(Showing off, boasting, exaggerating, praising. Vanity. Talking big)

Big, great   Breathing freely, (Talking, showing)

Hu

Tiger

Tiger's stripes   Person's legs

If we look beyond the dictionary meanings of the elements composing *kua* to see their images, we find a picture of a foot, representing movement, combined with a representation of great and free breathing. This suggests the feeling we all know after practicing Taiji for some time – of being carried along by the breath, of riding the Taiji energy.

This is our third encounter with *hu*. If we are thinking of Tiger as a metaphor for the Taiji energy, we can see our first meeting, in *Bao hu gui shan,* as the recognition of this energy within us and our ability to bring it into our center. And we can see the second meeting, in *Da hu,* as our learning to use it – in fighting, working, playing, and meditating – in everything we do. Now, with a shift in awareness, we *Kua hu.* Now we feel an intimacy with Tiger that allows us to let go enough to just go along for the ride. *Da hu* is about our doing Taiji. *Kua hu* is about Taiji doing us.

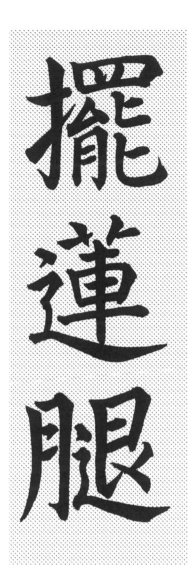

Bai lian tui

(by lyáhn tway)

Lotus kick 106

Bai

Placing, arranging, spreading, waving, swaying, shaking, moving, revealing, assuming. Pendulum . . . Hands catching a bear?

Hand

Bear captured in a net. (Stopping, finishing, resigning)

Net   Bear (Ability, skill)

Lian

Lotus . . . The plant with the wheel-like flower

Grass, herbs, weeds

Carriage rolling along. (Linking, joining, connecting, succeeding, repeating)

Tui

腿

Leg . . . Part of the body for walking

Flesh, parts of the body 月 艮 Person moving along, walking

Again we find the possibility of potent metaphor in the images making up these characters:

First there is *Bai,* which carries in its meaning a connotation of ordered movement. But what does a bear caught in a net have to do with this? Could it possibly be a reference to Ursa Major, the constellation which the Chinese, as well as we, know as the Great Bear of heaven? Ursa Major contains the Northern Dipper, the *Qi Xing* or seven stars (page 103), and we have learned that the Taoist movement meditation called Pacing the Dipper is also called Pacing the Network of Heaven. This constellation is definitely a symbol of rhythmic, ordered movement. The Great Bear is forever caught in the net that is the pattern of the stars, continually circling with the other constellations, revolving on the invisible wheel of the night and centered on the North Star – the still point, which represents the quiescence out of which enlightenment can flower.

Then we have that wheel-flower, the Lotus, the Golden Flower, organic symbol of the *light* of enlightenment and of the circle whose center is everywhere and whose circumference is nowhere.

This movement immediately follows our tiger ride, where we were aware of being carried along by, being *done* by, the Taiji energy. In the lotus kick, as we spin around our own center, our own still point, perhaps we can also experience, intuitively and immediately, our essential identity with the circling of heaven and the rhythms of nature. Perhaps the Golden Flower opens.

Lotus in the Manner of Xu Wei
Zhuda (c. 1626-1705) Qing dyn.
Hanging scroll: ink on paper, 1.850 x .898
Keith McLeod Fund. Courtesy, Museum of Fine Arts, Boston

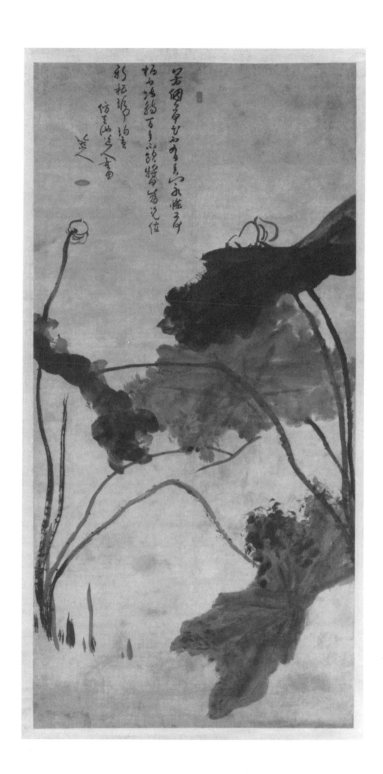

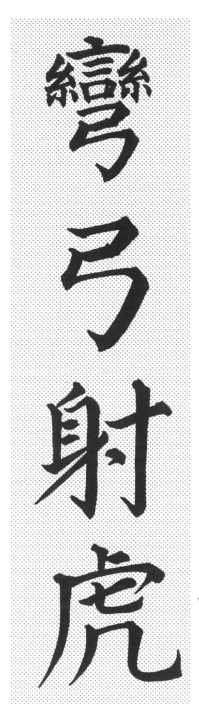

Wan gong she hu

(wahn gong shuh hoo)

Shoot tiger with bow   110

Wan

Bending, curving, flexing, turning . . . Pulling a bowstring

Bow   modern version of an ancient character showing a hand working with tangled threads. (Discord, trouble, quarreling)

Gong Bow

She

Shooting, aiming at . . . Shooting at a body with a bow

Body, person   Hand, which in the ancient character was an arrow

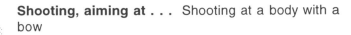

Hu Tiger

Tiger's stripes ... Person's legs

The last we saw of our tiger, we were sitting on top of it, and now here we are shooting at it. What happened? In the practice of archery as a meditation, the mind of the archer becomes one with the target. There is no separation, not even a thought, between them. There is only open awareness, making both aiming the arrow and hitting the target irrelevant. Purpose and goal disappear and only the spontaneous release, the letting go, remains.

Now we have gone beyond both *Da hu* and *Kua hu*. We are no longer doing Taiji and Taiji is no longer doing us, because we now are Taiji. The moment we shoot Tiger we release it as object, simultaneously releasing ourselves as subject. Self and other are not two. Perhaps we experience our own energy as not separate from, but identical to, the one, spiraling energy of the universe.

Once more we are reminded of Zhuangzi, who says that in the still-ness at the center of the circling there is no separation between This and That. In the center they are blended together in the infinite One and are seen as such in the Light. This somehow evokes an image of the self as a flashlight beam we can see when we project it into the dark, but which disappears in the full light of a sunny day.

While playing with these meanings, I discovered wonderful words written by Lu Xiangshan, founder of the Neo-Confucianist School of Mind in the twelfth century. He describes the indescribable – his enlightenment – in this way:

> "I raise my head and reach for the Northern Dipper. I spin around and live at the North Star. I hold my head high and see beyond Heaven. There is no such man as I."

How about that as support for intuitions about meaning in the last few names of Taiji movements? It is almost as if he is talking about those final movements: *Qi xing, Kua hu, Bai lian tui,* and *Wan gong she hu.* Could it be that Taiji is, after all, a movement allegory of the perpetual process of enlightenment?

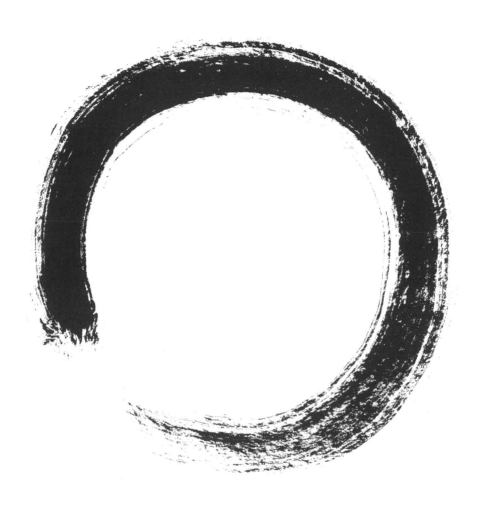

Calligraphy by Margaret Chang

The Tiger Way

So far in our game Tiger has been used as a symbol of the Taiji energy. But going along with the delightful ambiguity and poetry of the Chinese language and thinking, let's widen our vision to include another view of Tiger as metaphor. The basic process of this book clearly seemed to say: Tiger can represent any situation, any entanglement or attachment we encounter. And the Taiji form can represent a creative way of dealing with Tiger in this sense – a spiritual unfolding applicable to anything we do, from the most mundane to the most sublime.

Playing with the names of the Taiji movements seems to present to us a process we can call the Tiger Way. This Way is somewhat reminiscent of the Chan/Zen ox-herding pictures, but here we see five stages of this process instead of ten:

1. *Bao hu gui shan.* We embrace it. We discover something and claim it as our own, and/or perhaps it claims us as its own. We adopt it, and take it with us on our journey to the mountain top. Eventually we realize it may show us the way.

2. *Da hu.* We struggle with it. We interact with it. We learn what to do about, to, or with it. This involves gaining experience by participating. The practice of Taiji is about this – about learning a method based on the philosophy of Taoism. We recognize centeredness, balance and unity of body and mind. We learn to incorporate softness, fluidity and inner stillness into our Taiji and then into our lives. We learn the power of circling, yielding and harmonizing. Possibly we eventually realize our oneness with it, completing it and acquiring strength from it.

3. *Kua hu.* We ride it. We have tamed it, or perhaps it has tamed us. It is second nature now and we can let go of control. Where there was striving, there is now effortlessness. Perhaps this is what *Wu wei* is about – not doing, but being done. Now there is the potentiality of unity.

4. *Wan gong she hu.* We shoot it. If we reach this stage it is no longer second nature. It is our true nature and our true nature is it. We let go of the distinction between self and other, knower and known. Zhuangzi calls this the essence of Tao, when *this* is also *that* and *that* is also *this*. This stage is the pivot point – the still point around which all opposites spontaneously complete each other as they circle in harmony and unity.

5. *Bao hu gui shan.* We always embrace it again. We return to the beginning to repeat the process on another level. This is not a once and for all time thing, but ongoing and ever-expanding. And furthermore, the five stages can happen not only sequentially, but also randomly or simultaneously. It boggles the mind!

A Conclusion

So now it's time to shoot this tiger – this playing with the names of the Taiji movements. It's time to forget the words and return to the beautiful, silent movement, both of Taiji and Chinese calligraphy. For Taiji is not in the words about it, whether they are Chinese or any other language. It is not in the images. It is in the silent dance of body, mind and heart. Probably, the more we talk about it, the farther we stray from its meaning.

Let's return to Zhuangzi once more, to be reminded that after we catch the fish we can forget about the net. After we catch the rabbit we can forget about the trap. And after we catch the meaning we can forget about the words. "He who knows does not speak; he who speaks does not know."